Brought to you exclusively by

DTP
DIGITAL TO PRINT

GLUTEN FREE
LIVING

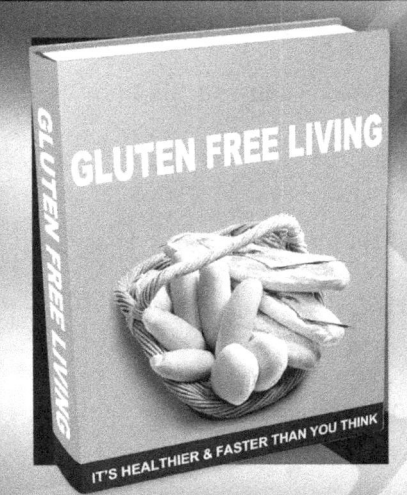

GLUTEN FREE LIVING

IT'S HEALTHIER & FASTER THAN YOU THINK

It's Healthier & Easier Than You Think!

GLUTEN FREE LIVING
It's Healthier & Easier Than You Think!

© D.T.P. Editorial, 2014
© Dennis S. Lewiston
Master Resell Rights

ISBN-13: 978-1500994495
ISBN-10: 1500994499

Copyright © 2014 All rights reserved.

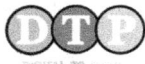

Table of Contents

CHAPTER 1

Introduction

A lifestyle that is healthy and promotes a good quality of life is important. As a parent, it is also one of the best gifts you can give to your children. Food is a necessity for our bodies to thrive but we live in a society were eating habits have moved in the wrong direction.

A lack of time, a lack of information, and the availability of processed foods has resulted in obesity, increased health risks, and reduced lifespan. These negative outcomes can make life difficult due to reduced energy, not being as alert, and an array of potential health problems.

If you are interested in making positive changes for yourself and for your household, consider the gluten free living option. You may be saying you are too busy for gluten free diet programs or that you will be limited in the foods you can buy.

However, this doesn't have to be the case. There are plenty of recipes and variety that are easy to make. There are more restaurants and grocery stores today that offer gluten free options than in the past. This is a lifestyle change that you will find there is a great deal of support surrounding and that makes it possible to successfully incorporate.

Until now, you may not have paid too much attention to gluten. Yet it is in so many of the foods that the average person eats without thinking twice about doing so. It seems to be everywhere you look now that you are making the effort to exclude it from your diet.

Instead of focusing on that negative fact though, focus on the positive changes you are going to make and the opportunity that you have to improve your overall well-being. As you learn more about gluten free products you can make better choices that help you.

Initially, a gluten free lifestyle may seem too hard to implement, but it doesn't have to be. Here, you will get the information you need about why you can live healthier and happier with this type of diet. You will find out methods for shopping and eating out that make it easier.

By eliminating the myths and sticking to the facts you can formulate your plan of action. You will get information about recipes, support, and the health benefits. As you read through the materials, you will be motivated to embrace such changes and you will have the methods to do so!

Not everyone out there is ready to act with a gluten free diet, and that is okay. Freedom of choice is very important. If you feel it is right for you than don't worry about what other people think. If you are friendly as you explain your reasons and while talking to those in a restaurant that are serving you then it isn't out of line at all.

In 2010, various research companies including the National Restaurant Association and American Culinary Federation named gluten free as one of the top food priorities to consider for their establishments. They realized this was more than a passing trend.

For millions of people, it has become a lifestyle choice that they engage in every single day. Are you ready to join them? It seems like all of the doors are wide open at this point when it comes to overall opportunity. The barriers that used to be in place such as limited products that were gluten free and a lack of information have been slowly removed.

Gluten problems can affect people of all ages, including children. There is no indication that any race or gender is more likely to be affected by it than others. The sooner that the problem is identified though the better.

Many adults develop this problem as they get older and there are a multitude of reasons why. There is nothing you can do to prevent it though as it is a genetic factor. You can take action though to live a good quality of life though in spite of the situation.

CHAPTER 2

What is Gluten Free Living?

Gluten is a type of protein that is found in various foods including rye, barley, and wheat. While most of us take for granted being able to digest this protein that isn't the case for millions of others. Instead, their body struggles with it every time they consume any gluten.

There are some individuals that have an adverse reaction to gluten so they must eliminate it from their body. Their body will actually fight digesting it as it is deemed as the enemy and the body is ready to attack. This is why it can lead to nutritious deficiencies and also to chronic fatigue. The body isn't able to use the nutrients taken in and so much energy is spent fighting the gluten.

However, many people decide to make such a change in order to feel better and to promote longevity. Many popular celebrities talk about their gluten free diet and that tends to get the attention of the average person as well.

Gluten free living means you no longer consume the foods that contain gluten in them. You do need to make sure you watch out for cross contamination issues that can occur. For example, oats don't have gluten in them but due to the way they are processed and packaged they should be assumed to have gluten in them unless the packaging for that particular product specifically states otherwise.

You will still get to consume a wide variety of foods though which is very important. No one wants to feel like they are strictly limited to just a few choices for their meals. There are gluten free main courses, side dishes, and even desserts you can enjoy. The food tastes great too so you aren't going to be settling for bland options or food that you have to force yourself to consume.

It is also important to know that a proper gluten free lifestyle offers your body the vitamins, minerals, and fiber that you need on a daily basis. A large portion of your diet will include fresh fruits and vegetables. If you already like to eat fruits and vegetables then this is going to be an easier lifestyle change for you than you might have thought.

They also offer your body powerful antioxidants to help remove toxins from your body. You will feel satisfied rather than hungry, provide your body with fuel, and have energy for your daily routine and exercise.

You may be fearful at first about a diet that is free from gluten but you will be very happy with the choices out there. You will find a variety of great foods and you can even have cake and other delicious items made with flour alternatives.

See your Doctor

It isn't recommended to self diagnose when it comes to a gluten problem. You should consult with your doctor to have the correct testing done. Some of the symptoms of gluten problems can be the same as other forms of health problems so it is important to get a professional diagnosis.

Continue to eat the way you normally would though when you are scheduled for the testing. If there is no gluten in your body then the blood work isn't going to be able to determine that it is the core of the problem (if indeed it is)! If your blood work shows that there is a problem then you can remove the gluten.

Of course if you are making the change because you want to and not because of a medical concern then you can make the change when you are ready. Either use up the items you have in your home with gluten or toss them out and make a fresh break from it. Many people find tossing those items in the trash is quite empowering!

The outreach in place for this type of testing has significantly grown in the past couple of years. Part of the education process involves getting more doctors to prescribe such testing for their patients. By 2019 the goal is to successfully diagnose as many cases as possible so that children and adults with a gluten concern aren't slipping through the cracks and increasing the risk of serious health problems.

Some individuals will still notice they have some symptoms even after they switch to a gluten free diet. This can be due to the severity of their condition. It can also be due to the damage that has occurred for the small intestine. While the small intestine is healing itself, your doctor may recommend that you take dietary supplements in order if malnourishment has occurred.

Many individuals that are changing to a gluten free diet aren't getting the amount of certain vitamins that their body needs. Your doctor may recommend a supplement to increase the amount of Vitamin B, iron, zinc, or calcium. If such supplements are recommended take them until your doctor feels you no longer need them.

Household Items to Watch for Most people have the understanding that gluten is only found in foods that you consume. However, there are some household items that may contain it so you need to be diligent in looking at them too. Here are the most common ones that you need to take a very close look at before you use them again. It will depend on the brand so you need to read the label:

- Chapstick
- Glue
- Gum
- Medicines (Including over the counter, herbal remedies, and prescriptions)
- Toothpaste

CHAPTER 3

Why is Gluten Free Living a Good Idea?

Some individuals have no choice but to follow a gluten free lifestyle due to the way their bodies process it. Celiac disease is a type of autoimmune disorder that results in the body rejecting gluten instead of processing it. The gluten is seen as a toxin to their bodies and it can create very serious health problems.

The severity of the reaction can vary based on the individual and the amount of gluten that they consume. A gluten allergy is extremely common, but it is very rarely diagnosed. Today, more people are informed about the symptoms and more medical professionals are testing for it.

This is why the number of children with sensitivity to gluten is being identified. There are adults that have struggled with their health for their entire life though because this gluten problem was never addressed. The sooner that a person is diagnosed though the sooner changes to their diet can be implemented.

It is believed that 1 in 133 people have some form of Celiac disease. The problem is that when they are consuming gluten their small intestine is being damaged. This creates problems with the small intestine successfully absorbing nutrients that the body needs. Some reports indicate approximately 83% of the cases though aren't diagnosed.

Celiac disease is genetic so if anyone in your family has it then your risk increases. Some individuals have several symptoms and others don't have any at all. There are more than 300 possible symptoms that can occur, but these are the most common:

- Abdominal pain
- Anemia
- Bloating
- Bone pain
- Chronic fatigue
- Depression

- Diarrhea
- Fertility problems
- Gas
- Headaches
- Weight changes

Children may have some other symptoms that develop including:

- Behavioral changes
- Dental enamel damage
- Distended abdomen
- Failure to gain weight or height at their percentile

In order to confirm such a diagnosis, blood work is completed. If it comes back positive, than a biopsy of the small intestine will be done to see if the lining has been damaged as well as the degree of any damage that has occurred. There is no cure for Celiac disease other than to follow a gluten free diet.

Doing so allow the small intestine to heal and in time it can allow a person to make a full recovery. Their body will start being able to use the nutrients that they consume for better overall health. The problem will get worse if dietary changes aren't made including malnutrition, osteoporosis, neurological problems, and Lymphoma.

Request testing for you and your children if possible because so many people go undiagnosed with this type of problem. If you think this could be the issue, don't want until your doctor brings up the idea of the testing. Ask your family members too in order to determine if there is a high chance of it occurring for you or your child.

Some individuals develop Dermatitis Herpetiformis, often referred to as DH, which is a type of Celiac disease that affects the skin. In order to diagnosis it blood work and a skin biopsy are conducted. The only cure for it is also a gluten free diet.

Such a test is a good ideas as this type of skin problem is often mistaken for Eczema. It can be very frustrating when the medication for Eczema is given but the condition either stays the same or gets worse. Until the diet is changed then the skin isn't going to clear up.

Many people make the choice to have a gluten free diet even though they don't have the disease. Some have a family history of many health problems and they are being as proactive as possible to reduce the risk of serious health concerns for them personally.

If you decide to make this your lifestyle due to your own personal beliefs, you need to stand up for it. Don't let others that don't agree with you or that don't understand your decision to create problems or doubts for you. Not everyone in your life will be supportive about it but the majority of people will.

A gluten free lifestyle isn't something to be shy about, to be ashamed of, or that you need to hide. It may be different from other people and the food choices they make but that is okay. It is about doing what is right for you and for your family in this regard so don't succumb to peer pressure.

Parents try to do all they can to create a world for their children that is fair, that is fun, and that is rewarding. Yet there can be issues with children that society as a whole isn't kind about. For example, children that have ADD or ADHD or those with Autism.

As the parent of a child with those types of issues, it can be exhausting. It can be hard for you and your partner to deal with on a daily basis. You may feel like you have been isolated by your friends and family because of it. Not giving up on your child though is important.

Some parents have found that their child did significantly improve by removing gluten from their diet. This was a better option or them than medicating their child. When there are behavior issues that aren't explained, it is definitely worth trying a gluten free diet for a few months and monitoring the behavior of your child.

If you see improvements, then that is encouraging and you should continue the diet. It could make a huge difference in the happiness of your child, in the dynamics of your household, and even how your child is accepted socially.

There are a few studies out there that indicate a gluten free diet can be a way to reduce symptoms of other forms of autoimmune deficiencies too. This includes:

- Cystic Fibrosis
- Multiple Sclerosis

- Thyroid Disease

Such information is very encouraging because it can be very upsetting to deal with the symptoms of these autoimmune deficiencies. They can create pain, fatigue, and other symptoms that affect every element of a person's life. If changing to a gluten free diet can make these health problems more manageable, isn't it worth it to consider?

Other individuals have taken on a gluten free lifestyle due to having a child or partner that needs to follow such a diet plan. It is certainly easier to create meals that everyone in the household can consume rather than making something different from the person that can't have gluten. Plus, if a parent has a gluten related issue that it is very possible children in the household will at some point. Teaching them a healthier way of eating from an early age is important.

There are people that choose not to consume gluten because they feel better removing it from their diet. While they didn't test positive for Celiac disease, they may have some sort of wheat allergy. They may have an intolerance or sensitivity to gluten.

They often have gas or bloating when they consume it so they have removed if from their diet to be more comfortable. They don't have damage to the small intestine due to the gluten but they just feel better overall by not consuming it anymore.

No one wants to try to get through their day continually with bloating and gas. It can make it hard to focus on work, social activities, and even intimate relationships. With the anxiety gone about such symptoms, it can give a person a refreshing and upbeat outlook about life that was missing before.

Weight loss and weight maintenance has also been a reason to stop consuming gluten. The craving for sweets can make it hard to stick to a good diet plan but many people find they don't have cravings after a few weeks of a gluten free diet.

They also find that they lose weight and keep it off because they are no longer reaching for foods that have empty calories or snacks that are processed. Such changes can also do wonders for the amount of energy a person has.

Many people feel that they have been on a losing course for weight loss for quite some time. They don't have the willpower to stick with a program that is restricting them and they really shouldn't. Fad diets may be very popular but they are really just setting people up to fail. Many people find that they can stick with a gluten free diet and that they do lose weight.

There are a few reasons for that to occur. As previously mentioned, the cravings go away and that makes selecting healthier choices easier. Reducing the amount of processed foods that are consumed means that there is less harmful carbs that the body will store as fat. There is also less sugar intake that will be stored as fat.

The increased energy with this lifestyle also gives someone that help them may need to really exercise. They may have had a hard time doing so before but now they have both the energy and the motivation to stick with a plan of action. As they feel better and their mood improves it becomes a path that they would like to continue going down.

The verdict is still out there by the experts though regarding recommending the gluten free diet for weight loss. Since it can't be proven without in depth and time consuming studies you won't find doctor's that readily recommend it. However, you will find plenty of people that state it was the change that allowed them to feel great and to drop the pounds when nothing else worked.

If you have hit a point where you feel like losing weight is a lost cause, you may wish to give this type of lifestyle a try for a 90 day period. If you find that you feel better, you have more energy, and that you have lost weight then it is an option to continue with it.

Regardless of your reason for deciding to follow a gluten free diet – by necessity or by choice – it doesn't have to be hard and it doesn't have to be time consuming. It doesn't mean that you have a huge grocery bill or that you can't enjoy going out to eat.

If you travel often, you may be worried but you can use the internet to help you find great menu choices and restaurants anywhere you may go that offer gluten free selections. You have the ability to make this work for you and all of the information you need is at your fingertips!

Children and Gluten Free Diets

If your child is following a gluten free diet – by necessity or by your parenting choice – talk to them about it. It is amazing what children can learn even from an early age about making good food choices. Explain to them the importance of their food choices.

Let them know that if they are in doubt about what they can eat then they should refrain from consuming it until they get approval from an adult. Make sure your child's gluten diet is well known when they go to stay with a friend too. You can talk to the parent's in advance to make accommodations.

Offer to send a gluten free meal and snacks so that they don't feel obligated to buy special items for your child to be a guest in their home. This also reduces the risk that they may not properly follow labeling due to not having enough information to make the right choices.

At the other end of that spectrum, think about elderly individuals you may be responsible for. If you make their meals or they are in an assisted care facility they may need a gluten free diet plan. Make sure anyone that is in charge of their care understands what they can eat and what they can't.

Exercise

It is very important to point out that daily exercise is important for people of all ages. Taking part in a gluten free diet is a step in the right direction for overall health, losing weight, and maintaining a healthy body weight. Exercise still needs to be a part of the daily routine. Many individuals didn't exercise enough before due to their diet.

They continually felt fatigued and sluggish so it was hard for them to take part in working out. Once they changed to a gluten free diet though they found that they were able to benefit from the additional energy. They were energetic all day long too without peaks and valleys in there that once required a sugar intake as a pick me up.

Talk to your doctor about starting any new exercise program. Keep in mind that if you make too many changes at once to your lifestyle it will be hard to stick with it. Focus on the dietary changes and becoming familiar with what you can eat and what you can't first.

Then as your energy level increases and you are getting comfortable with your dietary changes you can look at the exercise plan. Find forms of exercise you can take part in that are at your fitness level. You should also take part in forms of exercise that you will enjoy so you will stick with them.

CHAPTER 4

Shopping for Food & Eating Out

Planning your meals is an important part of a gluten free lifestyle. It reduces the need for you to make an unhealthy choice because you are pushed for time. Plan your snacks too so that you always have something you can reach for when you get hungry. You don't have to be overwhelmed by the task of going to the grocery store though.

There are more stores that offer gluten free products than you may realize. The demand for them as well as the variety of options continues to grow all the time. You can go online to find out where to shop locally for those items you want. If you aren't finding enough selection, talk to the manager.

They may be willing to add a few gluten free items to what they normally stock if customers ask for it. Studies show that as of 2012, approximately 15% of customers were shopping for only gluten free products. Up to 25% were buying products gluten free as they have scaled down on the volume of gluten that they consume.

The predictions from U.S. News and World Report is that this percentage is only going to continue to climb in the future. Retailers that sell groceries are certainly going to be paying attention to this information as well and preparing the shelves in their stores to meet that demand.

Being well informed is important when you are shopping for gluten free products. Some of the common foods you may normally reach for to add to your basket contain gluten including:

- Bagels
- Cereal
- Crackers
- Pasta
- Pizza

Identifying what you can safely eat and what you can't is important so that you can be a great shopper. To help you feel better about all of this, focus on what you can eat and not what you are giving up.

Remember the many health benefits that you will gain when you start to feel your willpower slipping. The more you shop for gluten free items, the easier it becomes. Soon, it will be second nature for you when you enter the store.

Carefully Read Labels!

Different brands of products can contain gluten or not so you need to become familiar with the products out there. Don't be in a rush when you shop so that you can take all the time you need to read labels. Some products say gluten free and others say low gluten.

Fruits and Vegetables

Any fresh fruits and fresh vegetables that you see in the grocery store aren't processed and they are gluten free. You can buy sweet potatoes and white potatoes as they don't contain any gluten either. Both dry beans and peas are acceptable.

Dairy

Just about all of the milk and cheese that you will find at the grocery store are free of gluten. There are some exceptions though so you need to carefully read labels. Some processed cheese products have wheat in them and blue cheese does. If you buy plain yogurt there is no gluten. However, if you buy various flavors then there can be so always check the labels.

Meat, Fish, Pork, & Poultry

Look for lean cuts of meat, pork, and poultry. Only buy fresh fish and other forms of seafood. When you are looking at canned or frozen products in this category, many of them can contain gluten due to the processing. Always take the time to carefully read the labels. When possible, use fresh products instead of frozen or canned as they are better for you.

Grains

Select grains that are free of gluten. You will find that you can pick the varieties you like too. There are gluten free options with white, brown, and wild rice so your choice won't be limited.

Dining Out

When it comes to dining out, spend some time looking online to identify which restaurants offer you such dishes. This is very important if you are traveling and aren't familiar with the area. With the technology today, you can use your smartphone or a laptop to see what is available where you happen to be.

If you aren't able to do that, ask when you arrive about any gluten free foods that they may offer. Some locations are willing to make something special for you. With more restaurants trying to appease the needs of everyone it is possible they will work with you. Try to arrive at off peak times so they can provide you with personalized service.

There are some common items you can get though that would be fine. For example, order chicken or fish with a side of vegetables. You can also get a baked potato and a salad. You may want to ask what type of oil that fish or chicken is cooked in though as some of them do contain gluten.

There is a great deal of gluten in various marinades and sauces. If you aren't sure they are free of gluten it is best to avoid them. You can ask for them to be put on the side and most restaurants will be happy to comply.

Don't expect there to be gluten free bread or crackers though so make sure you don't reach for them unless you are positive!

It is fine to consume champagne and wine as they are made from grapes. However, most beer is going to be off limits due to the grains they use to make them. You will find some gluten free beer offers though in many restaurants so it doesn't hurt to ask. You can also consider various forms of mixed drinks.

If dessert is something you just don't want to pass up, you aren't going to have to. There are some great choices in this category too. If the restaurant is gluten free friendly they may have flourless cake available. You can also consider sorbet, sherbet, fresh fruit, or ice cream. They are universal options so there is a very good chance they will be available.

Some labels on products aren't as clear as they should be when it comes to determining if they contain gluten or not. If that is the case with a particular product, err on the side of caution. Don't buy it and you can do some research at home about it. You can always buy that product on your next shopping trip if you do find it is actually free of gluten.

The more you are aware of what you can eat and what you shouldn't, the easier it is for you to shop and for your to dine out without stress or worry. See appendix 1 for a list to help you as you work to become more familiar with your options.

CHAPTER 5

Recipes

It is a good idea to add the following items to your shopping list and to keep them on hand in your kitchen. They are commonly called for in gluten free recipes. You can also use them when you run low on food items for your menu to make something.

- Gluten free baking mix
- Gluten free crackers
- Gluten free bread crumbs
- Gluten free flour
- Gluten free snacks
- Guar Gum
- Quinoa
- Rice (brown or white depending on your preference)
- Xantham Gum

With these items you can also use some of your favorite recipes but with a gluten free value to them. It can be both fun and productive to get creative with those recipes. Here are some great tips for starting with such replacements:

- Binders – Use Xanthan Gum, Guar Gum, or gelatin.
- Breading – Wheat or gluten free bread crumbs or crushed potato chips.
- Flour – Use gluten free flour mix or cornstarch. There are plenty of options to consider including amaranth and sorghum.
- Thickening – Use cornstarch or gluten free baking mix. For a sweet recipe, use dry pudding mix.

The internet is a wonderful resource for finding various gluten free recipes to try. You will enjoy the new tastes and you will gain more confidence in this lifestyle choice as you are able to create meals you and your family love. You can also buy gluten free cookbooks, magazines, or exchange recipes with others that are also eating gluten free.

Here are some great ideas to get you started. Try some new recipes and create a file for those that you really like. As your file grows you can ensure lots of variety in your diet so you don't feel restricted or bored by eating the same thing over and over again.

Breakfast Ideas

Yogurt is a great option but make sure it is gluten free as many varieties aren't. Both Stonyfield and Chobani are certified by the Gluten Intolerant Group. You can use the yogurt as a basis for a delicious tasting smoothie too.

There are various brands of gluten free cereal by General Mills and Nature's Path. If you like hot cereal consider Cream of Buckwheat. There are also oats that are certified to be gluten free. Eggs that are fried or scrambled are a great way to start the day due to the amount of protein they offer.

Lunch Ideas

Lunch meat is a great choice for a convenient and gluten free option, but make sure it isn't processed. A salad can be a choice that works for you due to all of the vegetables. You have to be careful though as some of the cheese items and various dressings can have gluten in them.

Nachos consisting of tortilla chips and some melted cheese that is gluten free is a change from your basic lunch and very appetizing. Peanut butter on gluten free bread is another great consideration.

Dinner Ideas

Lean cuts of meat including beef, pork, and poultry are great choices. You can also consume fresh fish or other seafood. Adding fresh vegetables and your choice of potatoes offers you a wonderful meal without gluten in no time at all. You can also replace the potatoes with your choice of gluten free rice.

Snack Ideas

Gluten free snacks you can enjoy between meals will keep you on track. Cut up fresh fruit and vegetables so you can grab them and go. You can pack them to take in the car or to have at your desk while working.

There are plenty of types of cheese that don't contain gluten, and they are wonderful for snacking. They also help you to get your calcium. With certain flavors of cheese you need to be careful as they can have some gluten in them so always read the packaging. Kids seem to really enjoy those individually wrapped cheese sticks.

While you should only consume chips in moderation, they are also gluten free when it comes to many varieties including most of those offered by Frito Lay. For a lower calorie snack consider popcorn. Make some hardboiled eggs and consume them when you need a snack. They will give you lots of energy.

Dessert Ideas

Both children and adults enjoy dessert, and you don't have to eliminate it due to a gluten free diet. Various brands of pudding are free of gluten and you will have a variety of flavors to pick from. Ice cream can also be a wonderful treat but you need to pay attention to the labels. So many ice cream varieties these days are packed with goodies so you need to pay attention to what is in there.

Cross Contamination

It is very important that you think about the risk of cross contamination in your own kitchen as well as those of others that prepare gluten free meals for you or your family. If the same tools are used to prepare such items as those that do have gluten then there can be some contamination.

Even a small amount of gluten can be dangerous to certain individuals so care has to be taken to prevent this. It is one more reason why changing the entire family to a gluten free diet may be the best option to consider.

Holidays

For many people, the holidays can be tough due to the restrictions of the diet. There can be parties to attend and various events where you have to be very careful about what you eat.

You may decide to make dinner at your own home and offer a gluten free meal for all. It is certainly an option to consider. Prepare yourself for the holidays and have a few items you can take along for snacks with you in case an event isn't gluten free friendly.

CHAPTER 6

Support

Your decision to be gluten free is one you should feel proud of no matter why you have made that decision. It is a good idea to get a support system in place as soon as you can about it. Share with your family, friends, and co-workers about your lifestyle change and what it entails. You will be pleasantly surprised at the many people that support you and even think about making the change for their own household.

Tell your healthcare providers about such changes too if they haven't mandated it due to a medical necessity. You will find that most medical professionals are very supportive of this type of dietary change.

Being well informed is important so you should consider magazines, books, and websites. However, you need to make sure you fully explore the credibility of such resources or you will end up with so much conflicting information it can make your head spin.

If you have questions, there are some very good organizations where you can direct your questions. They include the Celiac Disease Foundation and the Gluten Intolerance Group.

There are plenty of online forums where you can get support and meet new people. You may find it useful to be able to ask questions from those that are also going through similar changes in their lifestyle.

Being able to share recipes, to vent when you are discouraged, and even to be able to get some encouragement when you really need it is important. You can also offer support to others from time to time so it becomes a give and take.

Don't underestimate the value of this type of support as it helps to educate people about gluten free diets. The volume of the masses can also encourage more gluten free products in restaurants and grocery stores.

If you have children, make sure that their caregivers and teachers know they are on a gluten free diet. You may need to send your child with their lunch daily as the school or daycare lunch menu may not reflect this choice.

You may need to provide snacks too but if you feel this is the right method for your household then your caregiver and the school should work with you. Check to see if there are any gluten free cooking classes offered in your community.

This can be a great way to learn some new cooking methods, try some delicious recipes, and make some terrific friends that you can count on to help you as you help them get used to these dietary changes. You may find working with a dietician is useful as well.

CHAPTER 7

Conclusion

Depending on what you currently eat, changing to a gluten free lifestyle may be a moderate change or a significant change. With the right information, you can accept those changes and become well aware of what you can eat and what you need to steer clear of.

For many individuals, they find that they have already been consuming plenty of foods on this list. Increasing the volume of fresh fruits and vegetables that they consume while reducing the intake of processed foods is the best place to start. Take the changes one step at a time so that you can focus on them.

Educate yourself about the reasons why a gluten lifestyle is right for you and get support all around you where you can. Learn about the foods to eat, where you can shop locally, and even online providers that have free or low cost shipping on the items you can't find locally.

Find out about restaurants that offer gluten free meals as well as safe items you can get from standard restaurants. It is possible to live gluten free and to feel very good about your decision to do so. It doesn't have to be expensive and it doesn't have to be difficult.

The good news is that there is more awareness out there about it than in the past. More grocery stores and restaurants are embracing the needs of this sector of consumers. When it comes to what you eat, the choice is always yours.

However, many people in our society today don't eat what they should for their overall health and well-being. With a diet that consists of lots of processed foods you open up the opportunity for serious health problems that can reduce your quality of life and also your overall lifespan.

A gluten free diet isn't going to harm you like many fad diets will out there. This should be encouraging information if you are switching to this type of lifestyle because you want to rather than because you medically have to.

It is never too late to change your habits and start with a gluten free diet that works well for you. This type of diet can work for your entire family and they won't feel like they are missing out on anything! Consider such changes an investment in your quality of life, your longevity, and your opportunity to really lead by example for your children!

It is estimated by 2015 that there will be more than $5 billion annually for sales of gluten free products. This isn't a passing trend, this is a lifestyle change and a way of life for many people. The possibilities continue to grow and that makes it easier to embrace this type of living without difficulty and without it being an expensive endeavor.

Appendix 1

You don't want to be second guessing yourself all the time when it comes to eating gluten free. Getting it right is easier than you think once you learn the foundation of all of it. Don't worry, it will get easier and you will spend less time reading labels and conducting research as time goes by.

You can consume any gluten free grain products including:

- Amaranth
- Buckwheat
- Corn flour
- Cornmeal
- Grits
- Millet
- Montina
- Quinoa
- Rice (brown, white, enriched, or basmati)
- Sorghum
- Soy
- Vegetable oil

Common Staples:

- Cheese (most blends but read the labels)
- Beans

- Butter
- Lean meats
- Legumes
- Fresh fruit
- Fresh seafood
- Fresh vegetables
- Margarine
- Milk
- Yogurt (plain, read the labels on flavored)

Any of the following various ingredients:

- Annatto
- Dextrose
- Glucose Syrup
- Lactose
- Lecithin
- Malodextrin (it can be consumed even when it is made from wheat)
- Oat gum
- Silicon Dioxide
- Starch
- Surcose
- Vinegar (except malt vinegar)